The Super Tasty Keto Diet Recipe Book

Cheap and Simple Delicious Recipes affordable for Beginners

Otis Fisher

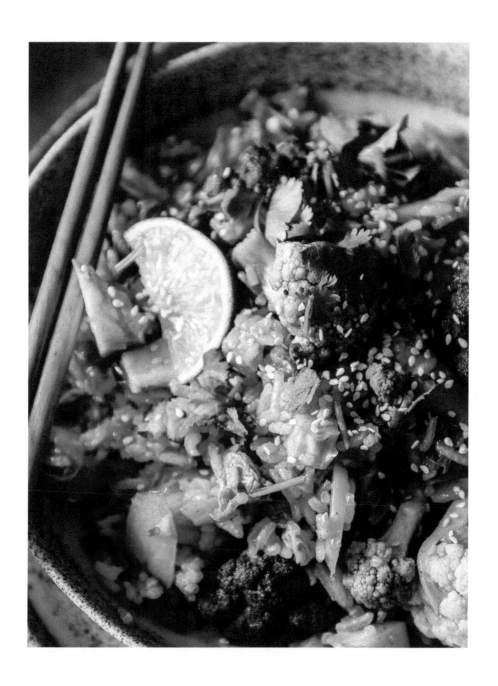

Please consult a licensed professional before attempting any techniques outlined in this book.

By reading this document, the reader agrees that under no circumstances is the author responsible for any losses, direct or indirect, which are incurred as a result of the use of information contained within this document, including, but not limited to, — errors, omissions, or inaccuracies.

Table of contents

Chaffles Ice cream Topping

Preparation Time: 7 minutes

Cooking Time: 5 minutes

Servings: 2

Ingredients:

- 1/4 cup coconut cream, frozen
- 1 cup coconut flour
- 1/4 cup strawberries chunks
- 1 tsp. vanilla extract
- 1 oz. chocolate flakes
- 4 keto chaffles

Directions:

1. Mix together all ingredients in a mixing bowl.
2. Spread mixture between chaffles and freeze in the freezer for 2 hours.
3. Serve chill and enjoy!

Nutrition:

Protein: 26

Fat: 71

Carbohydrates: 3

Easter Morning Simple Chaffles

Preparation Time: 7 minutes

Cooking Time: 5 minutes

Servings: 2

Ingredients:

- 1/2 cup egg whites
- 1 cup mozzarella cheese, melted

Directions:

1. Switch on your square Chaffle maker. Spray with non-stick spray.
2. Beat egg whites with beater, until fluffy and white.
3. Add cheese and mix well.
4. Pour batter in a Chaffle maker.
5. Close the maker and Cooking for about 3 minutes.
6. Repeat with the remaining batter.
7. Remove chaffles from the maker.
8. Serve hot and enjoy!

Nutrition:

Protein: 36

Fat: 60

Carbohydrates: 4

Low-Carb Bagels

Preparation Time: 15 minutes

Cooking Time: 30 minutes

Servings: 8

Ingredients

- 1/2 cup almond flour
- 1/4 cup coconut flour
- 1/2 Tbsp. psyllium husk
- 1 egg
- 1 egg white
- 2 Tbsp. coconut oil
- 2 Tbsp. coconut milk
- 1/2 Tbsp. apple cider vinegar
- 1/4 cup boiling water

Directions

1. Warmth the oven to 375F and line a baking sheet with parchment paper.
2. Whisk together the egg, egg white, apple cider vinegar, coconut milk, and coconut oil in a bowl.
3. Sift the rest of the ingredients in another bowl through a sieve.
4. Combine the two mixtures with a spatula and add boiling water.
5. Use your hands and roll the dough into 8 even balls.

6. Transfer the balls onto the baking sheet and flatten the dough to make the typical bagel shapes.
7. Place the sheet in the oven and bake for 30 minutes.
8. Cool and serve.

Nutrition:

Calories: 110

Fat: 8.6g

Carb: 6.4g

Protein: 3.2g

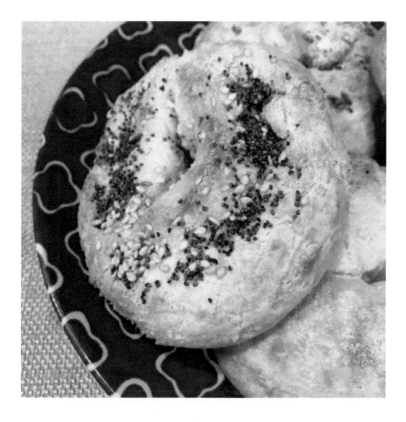

Cream Cheese Cookies II

Preparation Time: 10 minutes

Cooking Time: 10 minutes

Servings: 24

Ingredients

- 4 ounces butter, melted
- 2 ounces full fat cream cheese
- 1 egg
- 1-ounce coconut flour
- 1/2 tsp. baking powder
- 1/2 tsp. baking soda
- 1/4 tsp. liquid stevia extract
- 1/2 tsp. xanthan gum
- 1/2 tsp. vanilla extract

Directions

1. Preheat the oven to 350F. Line a cookies sheet with parchment paper.
2. Merge together the butter and cream cheese in a bowl.
3. In another bowl, mix the coconut flour, baking powder, xanthan gum, and baking soda.
4. In another bowl, add sugar substitute and vanilla to the egg and beat well.
5. Add the dry ingredients to the butter and cream cheese and mix well.

6. Stir in the egg mixture and combine everything well together.

7. Drop small spoonfuls of the mixture onto the prepared sheet and bake for 8 to 10 minutes.

8. Cool and serve.

Nutrition:

Calories: 51

Fat: 5g

Carb: 0.8g

Protein: 0.7g

Swiss Bacon chaffle

Preparation time: 10 minutes

Cooking Time: 8 Minutes

Servings: 2

Ingredients:

- 1 egg
- 1/2 cup Swiss cheese
- 2 tablespoons Cooked crumbled bacon

Directions:

1. Preheat your Chaffle maker.
2. Beat the egg in a bowl.
3. Stir in the cheese and bacon.
4. Pour half of the mixture into the device.
5. Close and Cook for 4 minutes.
6. Cook the second chaffle using the same steps.

Nutrition

Calories 23

Total Fat 17.6g

Saturated Fat 8.1g

Cholesterol 128mg

Sodium 522mg

Total Carbohydrate 1.9g

Dietary Fiber 0g

Total Sugars 0.5g

Protein 17.1g

Potassium 158mg

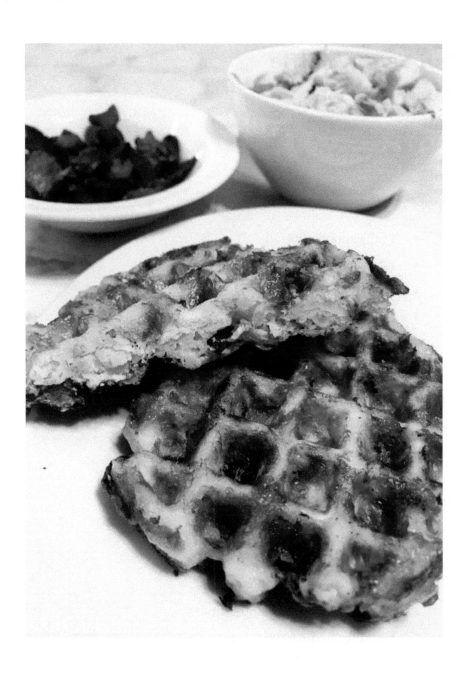

Chili Taco Chaffle

Preparation time: 8 minutes

Cooking Time: 20 Minutes

Servings: 2

Ingredients:

- 1 tablespoon olive oil
- 1 lb. ground beef
- 1 teaspoon ground cumin
- 1 teaspoon chili powder
- 1/4 teaspoon onion powder
- 1/2 teaspoon garlic powder
- Salt to taste
- 4 basic chaffles
- 1 cup cabbage, chopped
- 4 tablespoons salsa (sugar-free)

Directions:

1. Pour the olive oil into a pan over medium heat.
2. Add the ground beef.
3. Season with the salt and spices.
4. Cooking until brown and crumbly.
5. Fold the chaffle to create a "taco shell".
6. Stuff each chaffle taco with cabbage.
7. Top with the ground beef and salsa.

Nutrition

Calories 255

Total Fat 10.9g

Saturated Fat 3.2g

Cholesterol 101mg

Sodium 220mg

Potassium 561mg

Total Carbohydrate 3g

Dietary Fiber 1g

Protein 35.1g

Total Sugars 1.3g

Thanksgiving Keto Chaffles

Preparation time: 8 minutes

Cooking Time: 15 Minutes

Servings: 5

Ingredients:

- 4 oz. cheese, shredded
- 5 eggs
- 1 tsp. stevia
- 1 tsp. baking powder
- 2 tsp. vanilla extract
- 1/4 cup almond butter, melted
- 3 tbsps. almond milk
- 1 tsp. avocado oil for greasing

Directions:

1. Set eggs in a small mixing bowl; mix the eggs, almond flour, stevia, and baking powder.
2. Add the melted butter slowly to the flour mixture, mix well to ensure a smooth consistency.
3. Add the almond milk and vanilla to the flour and butter mixture, be sure to mix well.
4. Preheat Chaffles maker according to the manufacturer's instruction and grease it with avocado oil.
5. Set the mixture into the Chaffle maker and Cooking until golden brown.

6. Dust coconut flour on chaffles and serve with coconut cream on the top.

Nutrition

Protein: 3

Fat: 94

Carbohydrates: 3

Thanksgiving Pumpkin Latte with Chaffles

Preparation time: 10 minutes

Cooking Time: 5minutes

Servings: 2

Ingredients:

- 3/4 cup unsweetened coconut milk
- 2 tbsps. Heavy cream
- 2 tbsps. Pumpkin puree
- 1 tsp. stevia
- 1/4 tsp. pumpkin spice
- 1/4 tsp. Vanilla extract
- 1/4 cup espresso

For Topping

- 2 scoop whipped cream
- Pumpkin spice
- 2 heart shape minutes chaffles

Directions:

1. Mix together all recipe ingredients in mug and microwave for minutes Ute.
2. Pour the latte into a serving glass.
3. Top with a heavy cream scoop, pumpkin spice, and chaffle.
4. Serve and enjoy!

Nutrition

Protein: 16

Fat: 85

Carbohydrates: 10

Thanksgiving Pumpkin Spice Chaffle

Preparation time: 5 minutes

Cooking Time: 5minutes

Servings: 2

Ingredients:

- 1 cup egg whites
- 1/4 cup pumpkin puree
- 2 tsps. pumpkin pie spice
- 2 tsps. coconut flour
- 1/2 tsp. vanilla
- 1 tsp. baking powder
- 1 tsp. baking soda
- 1/8 tsp. cinnamon powder
- 1 cup mozzarella cheese, grated
- 1/2 tsp. garlic powder

Directions:

1. Switch on your square Chaffle maker. Spray with non-stick spray.
2. Beat egg whites with beater, until fluffy and white.
3. Add pumpkin puree, pumpkin pie spice, and coconut flour in egg whites and beat again.
4. Stir in the cheese, cinnamon powder, garlic powder, baking soda, and powder.
5. Set 1/2 of the batter in the Chaffle maker.
6. Close the maker and Cooking for about 3 minutes Utes.

7. Repeat with the remaining batter.
8. Remove chaffles from the maker.
9. Serve hot and enjoy!

Nutrition

Protein: 51

Fat: 41

Carbohydrates: 8

Triple Chocolate Chaffle

Preparation time: 5 minutes

Cooking Time: 7-9 Minutes

Servings: 2

Ingredients:

Batter

- 4 eggs
- 4 ounces cream cheese, softened
- 1 ounce dark unsweetened chocolate, melted
- 1 teaspoon vanilla extract
- 5 tablespoons almond flour
- 3 tablespoons cocoa powder
- 11/2 teaspoons baking powder
- 1/4 cup dark unsweetened chocolate chips

Other

- 2 tablespoons butter to brush the Chaffle maker

Directions:

1. Preheat the Chaffle maker.
2. Add the eggs and cream cheese to a bowl and stir with a wire whisk until just combined.
3. Add the vanilla extract and mix until combined.
4. Stir in the almond flour, cocoa powder, and baking powder and mix until combined.
5. Add the chocolate chips and stir.

6. Brush the heated Chaffle maker with butter and add a few tablespoons of the batter.

7. Close the lid and Cooking for about 8 minutes depending on your Chaffle maker.

8. Serve and enjoy.

Nutrition

Calories 385

Fat 33 G

Carbs 10.6 G

Sugar 0.7 G

Protein 12.G

Sodium 199 Mg

Walnuts Low carb Chaffles

Preparation time: 10 minutes

Cooking Time: 5 minutes

Servings: 2

Ingredients:

- 2 tbsps. Cream cheese
- 1/2 tsp. almonds flour
- 1/4 tsp. baking powder
- 1 large egg
- 1/4 cup chopped walnuts
- Pinch of stevia extract powder

Directions:

1. Preheat your Chaffle maker.
2. Spray Chaffle maker with Cooking spray.
3. In a bowl, add cream cheese, almond flour, baking powder, egg, walnuts, and stevia.
4. Mix all ingredients,
5. Spoon walnut batter in the Chaffle maker and Cooking for about 2-3 minutes Utes.
6. Let chaffles cool at room temperature before serving.

Nutrition

Protein: 12

Fat: 80

Carbohydrates: 8

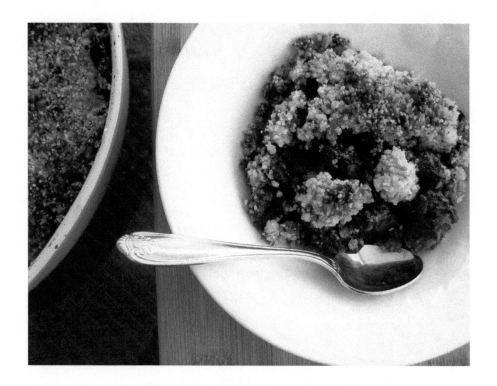

Yogurt Chaffle

Preparation time: 8 minutes

Cooking Time: 10 Minutes

Servings: 2

Ingredients:

- 1/2 cup mozzarella cheese, shredded
- 1/2 cup cheddar cheese, shredded
- 1 egg
- 2 tbsps. ground almonds
- 1 tsp. psyllium husk
- 1/4 tsp. baking powder
- 1 tbsp. Greek yogurt

Topping

- 1 scoop heavy cream, frozen
- 1 scoop raspberry puree, frozen
- 2 raspberries

Directions:

1. Mix together all of the chaffle ingredients and heat up your Chaffle Maker.
2. Let the batter stand for 5 minutes Utes.
3. Spray Chaffles maker with Cooking spray.
4. spread some cheese on chaffle maker and pour chaffle mixture in heart shape Belgian Chaffle maker.
5. Close the lid and Cooking for about 4-minutesutes.

6. For serving, scoop frozen cream and puree in the middle of chaffle.
7. Top with a raspberry.
8. Serve and enjoy!

Nutrition

Protein: 31

Fat: 66

Carbohydrates: 3

Zucchini Chaffle

Preparation time: 10 minutes

Cooking Time: 8 Minutes

Servings: 2

Ingredients:

- 1 cup zucchini, grated
- 1/4 cup mozzarella cheese, shredded
- 1 egg, beaten
- 1/2 cup Parmesan cheese, shredded
- 1 teaspoon dried basil
- Salt and pepper to taste

Directions:

1. Preheat your Chaffle maker.
2. Sprinkle pinch of salt over the zucchini and mix.
3. Let sit for 2 minutes.
4. Wrap zucchini with paper towel and squeeze to get rid of water.
5. Transfer to a bowl and stir in the rest of the ingredients.
6. Set half of the mixture into the Chaffle maker.
7. Close the device.
8. Cooking for 4 minutes.
9. Make the second chaffle following the same steps.

Nutrition

Calories 194

Total Fat 13 g

Saturated Fat 7 g

Cholesterol 115 mg

Sodium 789 mg

Potassium 223 mg

Total Carbohydrate 4 g

Crunchy Chaffle Cake

Preparation time: 2 minutes

Cooking time: 8 minutes

Servings 2

Ingredients:

- 1 egg
- 2 tablespoons almond flour
- 1/2 teaspoon coconut flour
- 20 drops Captain Cereal flavoring
- 1 tablespoon cream cheese
- 1/4 teaspoon baking powder
- 1/4 teaspoon vanilla extract
- 1/8 teaspoon xanthan gum
- 1 tablespoon butter, melted
- 1 tablespoon Swerve

Directions

1. Preheat the mini Chaffle maker.
2. Whisk all the ingredients until smooth and creamy in a large bowl. Allow the batter to rest for a few minutes.
3. Add about 2 to 3 tablespoons of batter to your Chaffle maker and cook for about 3 minutes. Repeat with remaining batter.
4. Serve immediately.

Nutrition:

Calories: 154

Fat: 11.2g

Protein: 4.6g

Carbs: 4.4g

Net Carbs: 2.7g

Fiber: 1.7g

Jicama Chaffle

Preparation time: 2 minutes

Cooking time: 8 minutes

Servings 4

- Ingredients:
- 1 large jicama root, peeled, shredded
- 2 eggs, whisked
- 1 cup shredded Cheddar cheese
- 1/2 medium onion, minced
- 2 garlic cloves, pressed
- Salt and ground black pepper, to taste

Directions:

1. Preheat the Chaffle maker.
2. Place shredded jicama in a large colander, sprinkle with salt. Mix well and allow draining. Squeeze out as much liquid as possible.
3. Microwave the salted jicama for 5 to 8 minutes.
4. Combine the jicama with the remaining ingredients in a large bowl.
5. Sprinkle a little more cheese on Chaffle maker before adding 3 tablespoons of the mixture, sprinkle a little more cheese on top of the mixture
6. Cook for 5 minutes. Flip and cook 2 minutes more.
7. Serve immediately.

Nutrition:

Calories: 168

Fat: 11.8g

Protein: 10.0g

Carbs: 5.1g

Net Carbs: 3.4g

Fiber: 1.7g

Cheesy Veggie Chaffle Stacks

Preparation time: 20 minutes

Cooking time: 14 to 18 minutes

Servings 2

Ingredients:

Fritters:

- 1 small zucchini
- ounces (150 g) frozen spinach, thawed and squeezed dry
- 1 large egg
- 1/4 teaspoon salt
- 1/8 teaspoon black pepper
- 1 tablespoon coconut flour
- 1 teaspoon onion powder
- 1/4 teaspoon garlic powder
- 1/8 teaspoon red pepper flakes
- 1/4 cup grated Parmesan cheese
- 2 teaspoons ghee

Mint Dressing:

- 1 tablespoon mayonnaise
- 1 teaspoon fresh lemon juice
- 2 tablespoons full-fat yogurt
- 1 tablespoon chopped fresh mint
- Salt and pepper, to taste

Directions:

1. Prepare a batch of the Basic Savory Chaffles by following the instructions of the first recipe. When done, set aside.
2. Make the veggie patties: Grate the zucchini and place it in a bowl lined with cheesecloth. Twist the cheesecloth around the zucchini and squeeze out the liquid out.
3. In a bowl, stir together the zucchini, spinach, egg, salt and pepper. Stir in the coconut flour and stir again. Add the onion powder, garlic powder, red pepper flakes and cheese. Mix until well combined.
4. Heat a large pan greased with the ghee over medium heat. Once hot, shape the mixture in to 2 large burgers and place them in the hot pan. Cook them until golden and crisp.
5. Make the dressing: In a small bowl, whisk together all the ingredients for the mint dressing.
6. Add a veggie patty on top of each chaffle. Drizzle each patty with the dressing and serve warm.
7. Secure in an airtight jar in the refrigerator for up to 3 days.

Nutrition:

Calories: 473

Fat: 36.8g

Protein: 25.2g

Carbs: 13.0g

Net Carbs: 7.7g

Fiber: 5.3g

Olive and Rosemary Chaffles

Preparation time: 10 minutes

Cooking time: 6 to 8 minutes

Servings 2

Ingredients:

Chaffles:

- 1 large egg white
- 1/2 cup grated Mozzarella cheese
- 1 teaspoon extra-virgin olive oil
- 2 tablespoons almond flour
- 2 tablespoons grated Parmesan cheese
- 1/4 teaspoon gluten-free baking powder
- Pinch of black pepper
- 6 Kalamata olives, pitted and sliced
- 1/4 teaspoon dried rosemary

Topping:

- 1 tablespoon extra-virgin olive oil
- 1/4 teaspoon minced garlic

Directions:

1. Preheat the Chaffle maker.
2. Combine the egg white, Mozzarella, and 1 teaspoon of the olive oil in a blender and blend until smooth. Add the almond flour, Parmesan, baking powder and black pepper.

Blend again. Add the olives and rosemary and stir them through.

3. Cook the batter: Follow the instructions of the Basic Savory Chaffles.

4. Make the topping: Mix the remaining 1 tablespoon of the olive oil and minced garlic and let it infuse while the chaffles are cooking.

5. Let the chaffles cool down slightly. Drizzle the garlic oil on top of the chaffles and serve.

6. Set in an airtight container at room temperature for up to 3 days, or in the refrigerator for up to 1 week.

Nutrition:

Calories: 250

Fat: 21.3g

Protein: 11.9g

Carbs: 3.6g

Net Carbs: 2.7g

Fiber: 0.9g

Strawberry Jelly Sandwich Chaffles

Preparation time: 10 minutes

Cooking time: 40 minutes

Servings 2

Ingredients:

- Strawberry Jelly (makes about 13 ounces / 369 g)
- 11/2 teaspoons gelatin powder
- 2 tablespoons water
- 12 ounces (340 g) fresh strawberries
- 1 tablespoon fresh lemon juice
- 3 tablespoons Swerve

Chaffles

- 4 Fluffy White Chaffles
- 1/4 cup roasted peanut butter
- 1/4 cup Strawberry Jelly

Directions:

1. To make the strawberry jelly, place the gelatin to a small bowl filled with 2 tablespoons of water. Leave to bloom for a few minutes. Set the strawberries in a blender and pulse until smooth.
2. Place half of the blended strawberries in a saucepan. Heat over medium-low heat and add the bloomed gelatin. Cook and stir until melted.

3. Remove from the heat and add the lemon juice, Swerve, and the remaining strawberries. Place in a jar and allow to cool. Once cool, transfer to the refrigerator for about 30 minutes.
4. To make the chaffles, prepare the Fluffy White Chaffles by following the instructions of the third recipe. Let them cool down completely.
5. Top two chaffles with peanut butter and strawberry jelly. Top each with the remaining chaffles and lightly press in.
6. Serve immediately.

Nutrition:

Calories: 232

Fat: 18.3g

Protein: 12.8g

Carbs: 8.1g

Net Carbs: 5.6g

Fiber: 2.5g

Pork Rind Chaffle with Marshmallow

Preparation time: 15 minutes

Cooking time: 20 minutes

Servings 2

Ingredients:

Chaffle Batter:

- 1 large egg
- 2 ounces (57 g) cream cheese, softened
- 1/4 teaspoon pure vanilla extract
- 1 ounce (28 g) pork rinds, crushed
- 2 tablespoons Swerve
- 1 teaspoon baking powder

Marshmallow Frosting:

- 1/4 cup heavy whipping cream
- 1/4 teaspoon pure vanilla extract
- 1 tablespoon Swerve
- 1/2 teaspoon xanthan gum

Directions:

1. Preheat the mini Chaffle maker.
2. In a medium mixing bowl, set together the egg, cream cheese, and vanilla.
3. Stir in the crushed pork rinds, Swerve, and baking powder to form a batter.

4. Add about 1/4 scoop of batter over the Chaffle maker. Cook for 3 to 4 minutes, then remove and cool on a wire rack. Repeat for remaining batter.

5. Meanwhile, whip the heavy whipping cream, vanilla, and Swerve until thick and fluffy. Sprinkle with the xanthan gum and fold until well incorporated.

6. Spread frosting over chaffles and cut, then refrigerate until set.

7. Serve chilled.

Nutrition

Calories: 334

Fat: 29.0g

Protein: 31.0g

Carbs: 24.0g

Net Carbs: 24.0g

Fiber: 0g

Broiled, Salted Pecans

Preparation time: 10 minutes

Cooking time: 6 to 8 minutes

Servings 2

Ingredients:

- 1 tablespoon (14 g) spread
- 1 cup (100 g) walnut parts salt

Directions:

1. Put the spread in a Pyrex pie plate and nuke on high for 30 seconds to dissolve. Include the walnuts and hurl until they're equally covered.
2. Set your walnuts back in the microwave and allow them 90 seconds on high. Mix and give them an additional 90 seconds to 2 minutes. Salt and eat up or keep in a snap-top compartment with a cover-for whatever length of time that you can stand up to.

Nutrition:

Calories 142

Fat 7.4 g

Carbohydrates 9.7 g

Sugar 3 g

Protein 9.g

Zucchini Olives Chaffles

Preparation time: 10 minutes

Cooking time: 15 minutes

Servings 2

Ingredients:

- Egg: 2
- Mozzarella Cheese: 1 cup (shredded)
- Butter: 1 tbsp.
- Almond flour: 2 tbsp.
- Turmeric: 1/4 tsp.
- Baking powder: 1/4 tsp.
- Onion powder: a pinch
- Garlic powder: a pinch
- Salt: a pinch
- Black pepper: 1/4 tsp.
- Spinach: 1/2 cup
- Olives: 5-10

Directions:

1. Boil the spinach in water for around 10 minutes and drain the remaining water
2. In a mixing bowl, add all the above-mentioned ingredients except for olives
3. Mix well and add the boils spinach
4. Pour the mixture to the lower plate of the Chaffle maker and spread it evenly to cover the plate properly

5. Sprinkle the sliced olives as per choice over the mixture and close the lid

6. Cook for at least 4 minutes to get the desired crunch

7. Remove the chaffle from the heat

8. Make as many chaffles as your mixture and Chaffle maker allow

9. Serve hot and enjoy!

Nutrition:

Calories: 121kcal

Carbohydrates: 3g

Protein: 9g

Fat: 8g

Cauliflower Mozzarella Chaffle

Preparation time: 10 minutes

Cooking time: 15 minutes

Servings 2

Ingredients:

- Cauliflower: 1 cup
- Egg: 2
- Mozzarella cheese: 1 cup and 4 tbsp.
- Tomato sauce: 6 tbsp.
- Basil: 1/2 tsp.
- Garlic: 1/2 tbsp.
- Butter: 1 tsp.

Directions:

1. In a pan, add butter and include small pieces of cauliflower to it
2. Stir for two minutes and then add garlic and basil
3. Set aside the cooked cauliflower
4. Preheat the mini Chaffle maker if needed
5. Mix cooked cauliflower, eggs, and 1 cup mozzarella cheese properly
6. Spread it to the mini Chaffle maker thoroughly
7. Cook for 4 minutes or till it turns crispy and then remove it from the Chaffle maker
8. Make as many mini chaffles as you can

9. Now in a baking tray, line these mini chaffles and top with the tomato sauce and grated mozzarella cheese
10. Put the tray in the oven at 400 degrees until the cheese melts
11. Serve hot

Nutrition:

Protein: 52

Fat: 39

Carbohydrates: 9

Plain Artichoke Chaffle

Preparation time: 10 minutes

Cooking time: 15 minutes

Servings 2

Ingredients:

- Artichokes: 1 cup chopped
- Egg: 1
- Mozzarella Cheese: 1/2 cup (shredded)
- Cream cheese: 1 ounce
- Salt: as per your taste
- Garlic powder: 1/4 tsp.

Directions:

1. Preheat a mini Chaffle maker if needed and grease it
2. In a mixing bowl, attach all the ingredients
3. Mix them all well
4. Pour the mixture to the lower plate of the Chaffle maker and spread it evenly to cover the plate properly
5. Close the lid
6. Cook for at least 4 minutes to get the desired crunch
7. Remove the chaffle from the heat and keep aside for around one minute
8. Make as many chaffles as your mixture and Chaffle maker allow
9. Serve hot with your favorite keto sauce

Nutrition:

Protein: 26

Fat: 71

Carbohydrates: 3

BBQ Sauce Pork Chaffle

Preparation Time: 5 minutes

Cooking Time: 15 minutes

Serving: 4

Ingredients:

- 1/2 pound ground pork
- 3 eggs
- 1 cup grated mozzarella cheese
- Salt and pepper to taste
- 1 clove garlic, minced
- 1 teaspoon dried rosemary
- 3 tablespoons sugar-free BBQ sauce
- 2 tablespoons butter to brush the Chaffle maker
- 1/2 pound pork rinds for serving
- 1/4 cup sugar-free BBQ sauce for serving

Directions

1. Preheat the Chaffle maker.
2. Add the ground pork, eggs, mozzarella, salt and pepper, minced garlic, dried rosemary, and BBQ sauce to a bowl.
3. Mix until combined.
4. Brush the heated Chaffle maker with butter and add a few tablespoons of the batter.
5. Close the lid and Cooking for about 7–8 minutes depending on your Chaffle maker.

6. Serve each chaffle with some pork rinds and a tablespoon of BBQ sauce.

Nutrition

Calories 350

Fat 21.1 g

Carbs 2.7 g

Sugar 0.3 g,

Protein 36.9 g

Sodium 801 Mg

Rosemary Pork Chops on Chaffle

Preparation Time: 5 minutes

Cooking Time: 15 minutes

Serving: 4

Ingredients:

- 4 eggs
- 2 cups grated mozzarella cheese
- Salt and pepper to taste
- Pinch of nutmeg
- 2 tablespoons sour cream
- 6 tablespoons almond flour
- 2 teaspoons baking powder

Pork chops

- 2 tablespoons olive oil
- 1 pound pork chops
- Salt and pepper to taste
- 1 teaspoon freshly chopped rosemary

Other

- 2 tablespoons Cooking spray to brush the Chaffle maker
- 2 tablespoons freshly chopped basil for decoration

Directions

1. Preheat the Chaffle maker.
2. Add the eggs, mozzarella cheese, salt and pepper, nutmeg, sour cream, almond flour and baking powder to a bowl.

3. Mix until combined.
4. Brush the heated Chaffle maker with Cooking spray and add a few tablespoons of the batter.
5. Close the lid and Cooking for about 5-7 minutes depending on your Chaffle maker.
6. Meanwhile, heat the butter in a nonstick grill pan and season the pork chops with salt and pepper and freshly chopped rosemary.
7. Cooking the pork chops for about 4–5 minutes on each side.
8. Serve each chaffle with a pork chop and sprinkle some freshly chopped basil on top.

Nutrition

Calories 66

Fat 55.2 g

Carbs 4.8 g

Sugar 0.4 g,

Protein 37.5 g

Sodium 235 Mg

Pork Loin Chaffle Sandwich

Preparation Time: 5 minutes

Cooking Time: 15 minutes

Serving: 4

Ingredients:

- 4 eggs
- 1 cup grated mozzarella cheese
- 1 cup grated parmesan cheese
- Salt and pepper to taste
- 2 tablespoons cream cheese
- 6 tablespoons coconut flour
- 2 teaspoons baking powder
- 2 tablespoons olive oil
- 1 pound pork loin
- Salt and pepper to taste
- 2 cloves garlic, minced
- 1 tablespoon freshly chopped thyme
- 2 tablespoons Cooking spray to brush the Chaffle maker
- 4 lettuce leaves for serving
- 4 slices of tomato for serving
- 1/4 cup sugar-free mayonnaise for serving

Directions

1. Preheat the Chaffle maker.

2. Add the eggs, mozzarella cheese, parmesan cheese, salt and pepper, cream cheese, coconut flour and baking powder to a bowl.
3. Mix until combined.
4. Brush the heated Chaffle maker with Cooking spray and add a few tablespoons of the batter.
5. Close the lid and Cooking for about 5–7 minutes depending on your Chaffle maker.
6. Meanwhile, heat the olive oil in a nonstick frying pan and season the pork loin with salt and pepper, minced garlic and freshly chopped thyme.
7. Cooking the pork loin for about 5–7 minutes on each side.
8. Cut each chaffle in half and add some mayonnaise, lettuce leaf, tomato slice and sliced pork loin on one half.
9. Cover the sandwich with the other chaffle half and serve.

Nutrition

Calories 710

Fat 52.7 g

Carbs 11.3 g

Sugar 0.8 g,

Protein 47.4 g

Sodium 513 Mg

Boiled Chicken Halloumi Chaffle

Preparation Time: 5 minutes

Cooking Time: 25 minutes

Servings: 2

Ingredients

- Boiled chicken: 1 cup shredded
- Pepper: 1/2 tsp.
- Salt: a pinch
- Halloumi cheese: 3 oz.
- Oregano: 1 tbsp.

Directions:

1. Take a bowl and add chicken, pepper, and salt
2. Make 1/2 inch thick slices of Halloumi cheese and divide each further into two
3. Put one slice of cheese in the unheated Chaffle maker and spread chicken on it
4. Top with another cheese slice and sprinkle oregano
5. Cooking the cheese for over 4-6 minutes till it turns golden brown
6. Remove from heat when a bit cool and serve with your favorite sauce

Nutrition:

Serving: 1g

Calories: 136

Carbohydrates: 2g

Protein: 10g

Fat: 10g

Sautéed Chicken Chaffle

Preparation Time: 5 minutes

Cooking Time: 25 minutes

Servings: 4

Ingredients

- Cheddar cheese: 1/3 cup
- Egg: 1
- Chicken: 2 small pieces sautéed in butter
- Baking powder: 1/4 teaspoon
- Salt: 1/4 tsp.
- Yogurt: 2 tbsp.
- Mozzarella cheese: 1/3 cup

Directions:

1. Mix cheddar cheese, egg, yogurt, chicken, baking powder, and salt together
2. Preheat your Chaffle iron and grease it
3. In your mini Chaffle iron, shred half of the mozzarella cheese
4. Add the mixture to your mini Chaffle iron
5. Again shred the remaining mozzarella cheese on the mixture
6. Cooking till the desired crisp is achieved
7. Make as many chaffles as your mixture and Chaffle maker allow

Nutrition:

Calories: 153

Fat: 12.2g

Carbohydrates: 0.7g

Sugar: 0.4g

Protein: 10.3g

Peppery Chicken Chaffles

Preparation Time: 5 minutes

Cooking Time: 25 minutes

Servings: 2

Ingredients

- Egg: 1
- Mozzarella Cheese: 1/2 cup (shredded)
- Boiled Chicken: 1/2 cup shredded
- Garlic powder: 1/2 tsp.
- Pepper: 1/4 tsp.
- Salt: 1/4 tsp.
- Dried basil: 1/2 tsp.

For Baking:

- Red Bell Pepper: 1 large thickly sliced
- Mozzarella cheese: 1/2 cup (shredded)
- Oregano: 1/2 tsp.

Directions:

1. Preheat a mini Chaffle maker if needed and grease it
2. In a mixing bowl, attach all the ingredients of the chaffle and mix well
3. Pour the mixture to the Chaffle maker
4. Cooking for at least 4 minutes to get the desired crunch and make as many chaffles as your batter allows
5. Preheat the oven

6. Spread chaffles on the baking sheet and top one pepper slice

7. Sprinkle cheese on top and put the baking sheet into the oven

8. Heat for 5 minutes to melt the cheese

9. Spread oregano on top and serve hot

Nutrition:

Carbs 8 g

Fat 11 g

Protein 5 g

Calories 168

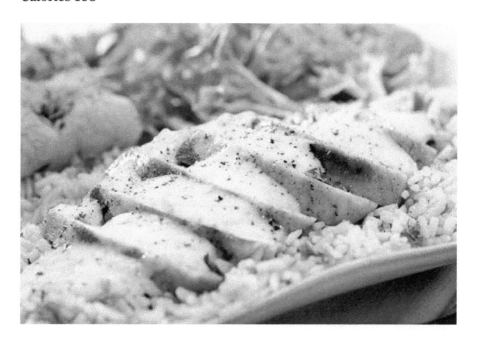

Sautéed Chicken Layered Chaffles

Preparation Time: 5 minutes

Cooking Time: 25 minutes

Servings: 2

Ingredients

- Chicken boneless: 1 cup sautéed in butter
- Egg: 2
- Mozzarella Cheese: 1 cup (shredded)
- Butter: 1 tbsp.
- Turmeric: 1/4 tsp.
- Baking powder: 1/4 tsp.
- Onion powder: a pinch
- Garlic powder: a pinch
- Salt: a pinch

Directions:

1. Mix all the remaining ingredients well together except the mince
2. Pour a thin layer on a preheated Chaffle iron
3. Add a layer of chicken mince on the mixture
4. Again add more mixture over the top
5. Cooking the chaffle for around 5 minutes
6. Serve hot with your favorite keto sauce

Nutrition:

Calories: 91

Fat: 5.9g

Carbohydrates: 0.3g

Sugar: 0.2g

Protein: 9.2g

Almond Chaffle Mix

Preparation Time: 5 minutes

Cooking Time: 10 minutes

Servings: 5

Ingredients

- 4 cups almond flour
- 2 cups almond milk
- 1/4 cup toasted wheat germ
- 1/4 cup toasted oat bran
- 1 cup buttermilk blend powder
- 3 tablespoons baking powder
- 2 teaspoons baking soda
- 1 teaspoon salt
- 1/2 cup mozzarella cheese, shredded
- 2 eggs
- 1 cup water
- 2 tablespoons canola oil
- 1 tablespoons honey

Directions:

1. In a bowl, set the first nine ingredients.
2. Set in an airtight container in the refrigerator for up to 6 months.
3. Yield: 8-1/2 cups mix (about 4 batches).
4. To prepare chaffles:
5. Place 2 cups Chaffle mix in a bowl.

6. Combine the eggs, water, oil and honey.
7. Stir into Chaffle mix just until moistened.
8. Set in a preheated Chaffle iron according to manufacturer's directions until golden brown.

Nutrition:

Calories 284,

Total Fat 19 g,

Cholesterol 89 mg,

Sodium 482 mg,

Total Carbohydrate 11 g,

Protein 15 g,

Fiber 5 g

Cinnamon Pecan Chaffles

Preparation Time: 1 hour 20 minutes

Cooking Time: 20 minutes

Serving: 5

Ingredients:

- 1 Tbsp. butter
- 1 egg
- 1/2 tsp. vanilla
- 2 Tbsp. almond flour
- 1 Tbsp. coconut flour
- 1/8 tsp. baking powder
- 1 Tbsp. monk fruit
- For the crumble:
- 1/2 tsp. cinnamon
- 1 Tbsp. melted butter
- 1 tsp. monk fruit
- 1 Tbsp. chopped pecans

Directions

1. Turn on Chaffle maker to heat and oil it with Cooking spray.
2. Melt butter in a bowl, and then mix in the egg and vanilla.
3. Mix in remaining chaffle ingredients.
4. Combine crumble ingredients in a separate bowl.
5. Pour half of the chaffle mix into Chaffle maker.
6. Top with half of crumble mixture.
7. Cooking for 5 minutes, or until done.

8.   Repeat with the other half of the batter.

Nutrition:

Calories: 101

Net Carb: 1.6g

Fat: 7.1g

Carbohydrates: 2.9g

Dietary Fiber: 1.3g

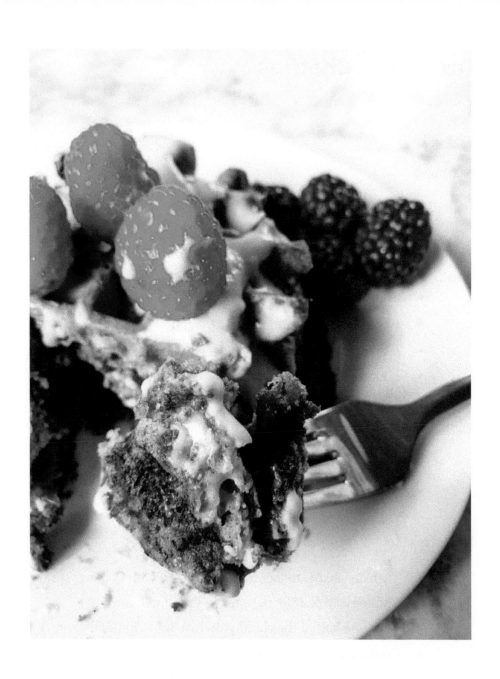

Oreo Keto Chaffles

Preparation Time: 5 minutes

Cooking Time: 6 minutes

Serving: 2

Ingredients:

- 1 egg
- 11/2 Tbsp. unsweetened cocoa
- 2 Tbsp. lakanto monk fruit, or choice of sweetener
- 1 Tbsp. heavy cream
- 1 tsp. coconut flour
- 1/2 tsp. baking powder
- 1/2 tsp. vanilla

For the cheese cream:

- 1 Tbsp. lakanto powdered sweetener
- 2 Tbsp. softened cream cheese
- 1/4 tsp. vanilla

Directions

1. Turn on Chaffle maker to heat and oil it with Cooking spray.
2. Combine all chaffle ingredients in a small bowl.
3. Pour one half of the chaffle mixture into Chaffle maker.
4. Cooking for 3-5 minutes.
5. Remove and repeat with the second half if the mixture.
6. Let chaffles sit for 2-3 to crisp up.
7. Combine all cream ingredients and spread on chaffle when they have cooled to room temperature.

Nutrition:

Calories: 98

Net Carb: 1.4g

Fat: 7.1g

Carbohydrates: 2.2g

Dietary Fiber: 0.8g

Keto Gingerbread Chaffle

Preparation Time: 5 minutes

Cooking Time: 6 minutes

Serving: 2

Ingredients:

- 1/2 cup mozzarella cheese grated
- 1 medium egg
- 1/2 tsp. baking powder
- 1 tsp. Erythritol powdered
- 1/2 tsp. ground ginger
- 1/4 tsp. ground nutmeg
- 1/2 tsp. ground cinnamon
- 1/8 tsp. ground cloves
- 2 Tbsp. almond flour
- 1 cup heavy whipped cream
- 1/4 cup keto-friendly maple syrup

Directions

1. Turn on Chaffle maker to heat and oil it with Cooking spray. Beat egg in a bowl.
2. Add flour, mozzarella, spices, baking powder, and Erythritol. Mix well.
3. Spoon one half of the batter into Chaffle maker and spread out evenly.
4. Close and Cooking for 5 minutes.
5. Remove cooked chaffle and repeat with remaining batter.

6. Serve with whipped cream and maple syrup.

Nutrition

Calories: 431 kcal

Carbohydrates: 6 g net

Protein: 16 g

Fat: 38 g

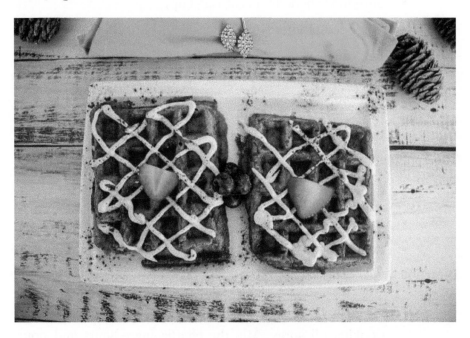

Raspberry Taco Chaffle

Preparation Time: 5 minutes

Cooking Time: 16 minutes

Serving: 1

Ingredients:

- Shredded cheddar cheese (.25 cup)
- Shredded Monterey jack cheese (.25 cup)
- Egg white (1)
- Coconut flour (1 tsp.)
- Stevia (.5 tsp.)
- Baking powder (.25 tsp.)

The Topping:

- Coconut flour (2 tbsp.)
- Raspberries (4 oz.)
- Raspberry sauce (2 oz.)

Directions:

1. Start the round Chaffle maker to preheat. Spray it using a Cooking oil spray. Mix the chaffle ingredients and pour them into the Cooker. Cooking it for 3-4 minutes.
2. Dip the raspberries in sauce and arrange them over the chaffle. Dust with the coconut flour and serve.

Nutrition:

Calories: 101

Net Carb: 1.6g

Fat: 7.1g

Carbohydrates: 2.9g

Coco-Kiwi Chaffles

Preparation Time: 5 minutes

Cooking Time: 16 minutes

Serving: 4

Ingredients:

- Cheddar cheese: 1/3 cup
- Egg: 1
- Kiwi: 1/2 cup finely grated
- Coconut flour: 2 tbsp.
- Baking powder: 1/4 teaspoon
- Coconut flakes: 2 tbsp.
- Mozzarella cheese: 1/3 cup

Directions:

1. Mix cheddar cheese, egg, coconut flour, coconut flakes, kiwi, and baking powder together in a bowl
2. Preheat your Chaffle iron and grease it
3. In your mini Chaffle iron, shred half of the mozzarella cheese
4. Add the mixture to your mini Chaffle iron
5. Again shred the remaining mozzarella cheese on the mixture
6. Cook till the desired crisp is achieved
7. Make as many chaffles as your mixture and Chaffle maker allow

Nutrition

Calories: 302 kcal

Carbohydrates: 12 g

Protein: 8 g

Fat: 27 g

Sugar: 6 g

Italian Seasoning Chaffles

Preparation time: 6 minutes

Cooking Time: 8 Minutes

Servings: 2

Ingredients:

- 1/2 cup Mozzarella cheese, shredded
- 1 tablespoon Parmesan cheese, shredded
- 1 organic egg
- 3/4 teaspoon coconut flour
- 1/4 teaspoon organic baking powder
- 1/8 teaspoon Italian seasoning
- Pinch of salt

Directions:

1. Preheat a mini Chaffle iron and then grease it.
2. In a container, add all ingredients and with a fork, mix until well combined.
3. Add half of the mixture into preheated Chaffle iron and Cooking for about 4 minutes or until golden brown.
4. Repeat with the remaining mixture.
5. Serve warm.

Nutrition:

Calories: 8et

Carb: 1.9g

Fat: 5g

Saturated Fat: 2.6g

Carbohydrates: 3.8g

Dietary Fiber: 1.9g

Sugar: 0.6g

Protein: 6.5g

Coconut Chaffles with Mint Frosting

Preparation Time: 15 minutes

Cooking Time: 28 minutes

Servings: 4

Ingredients

For the chaffles:

- 2 eggs, beaten
- 2 tbsp. cream cheese, softened
- 1 cup finely grated Monterey Jack cheese
- 2 tbsp. coconut flour
- 1/4 tsp. baking powder
- 1 tbsp. unsweetened shredded coconut
- 1 tbsp. walnuts, chopped

For the frosting:

- 1/4 cup unsalted butter, room temperature
- 3 tbsp. almond milk
- 1 tsp. mint extract
- 2 drops green food coloring
- 3 cups swerve confectioner's sugar

Directions

For the chaffles:

1. Preheat the Chaffle iron.
2. Incorporate all the ingredients for the chaffles.

3. Open the iron and add a quarter of the mixture. Close and cook until crispy, 7 minutes.

4. Transfer the chaffle to a plate and make 3 more with the remaining batter.

For the frosting:

1. In a medium bowl, cream the butter using an electric hand mixer until smooth.

2. Gradually mix in the almond milk until smooth.

3. Add the mint extract and green food coloring; whisk until well combined.

4. Finally, mix in the swerve confectioner's sugar a cup at a time until smooth.

5. Layer the chaffles with the frosting.

6. Slice and serve afterward.

Nutrition:

Calories 141

Fats 13.13g

Protein 4.31g

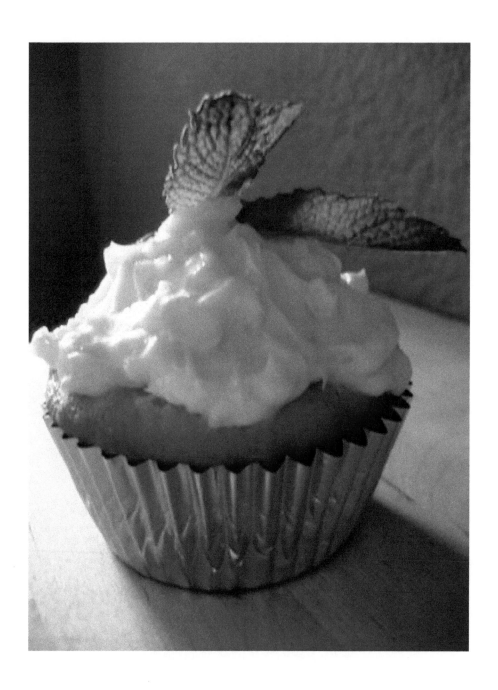

Keto Protein Chaffles

Preparation time: 40 minutes

Cooking time: 15 minutes

Servings: 11

Ingredients

- 5 pieces size M eggs
- 100 grams of pea protein I take this because it has low carbohydrates: pea protein
- 100 grams of cream
- 3 grams of baking powder
- 30 grams of butter
- 100 grams of mineral water
- 60 grams of almond cream
- 75 grams of stevia Erythritol I'll take this: Erythritol + stevia
- 15 grams of Amaretto Aroma

Directions:

1. Separate egg white and egg yolk.
2. Put all ingredients except the egg white in the bowl and stir.
3. Keto-protein chaffles-2
4. Beat the egg white into egg whites and fold in carefully.
5. Bake the Chaffles in the chaffle iron.

Nutrition:

Calories: 150

Net Carb: 0.

Fat: 11.9g

Saturated Fat: 6.7g

Carbohydrates: 0.6g

Coconut Cookies

Preparation Time: 10 minutes

Cooking Time: 7 minutes

Servings: 12

Ingredients

- 2 egg whites
- 1 1/2 cups coconut flakes
- 2 oz. butter, melted, cooled
- 2 Tbsp. coconut flour
- 1/4 cup Erythritol

Directions

1. Combine flour, coconut flakes, and Erythritol.
2. Add egg whites and melted butter. Mix.
3. Set a baking sheet with parchment paper and put the cookies batter on it by the spoonful.
4. Bake at 350F for 7 minutes.
5. Enjoy.

Nutrition:

Calories: 144

Fat: 10.4g

Carb: 7g

Protein: 1.4g

Keto Snicker doodle Chaffle

Preparation time: 5 minutes

Cooking time: 10 minutes

Servings: 2

Ingredients:

- 1 Egg
- 1/2 cup of Mozzarella Cheese
- 2 tbsp. Almond Flour
- 1 tbsp. Lakanto Golden Sweetener
- 1/2 tsp. Extract of Vanilla
- 1/4 tsp. Cinnamon
- 1/2 tsp. Baking Powder
- 1/4 tsp. Cream of tartar

Coating

- 1 tbsp. Butter
- 2 tbsp. Lakanto Classic Sweetener
- 1/2 tsp. Cinnamon

Directions:

1. Heat your mini Chaffle maker.
2. Mix all chaffle ingredients in a shallow mixing bowl.
3. Set half of the chaffle batter into the Chaffle irons middle. Allow for 3-5 minutes of Cooking time.
4. Remove carefully and repeat with the second chaffle. Allow chaffles to cool completely before serving.

5. To coat the sweetener, mix it with the cinnamon in a shallow bowl.

6. Brush the chaffles with butter that has been melted in a shallow microwave-safe bowl.

7. After brushing the chaffles with butter, sprinkle the sweetener and cinnamon mixture on both sides.

Nutrition:

CALORIES: 182

Total fat: 13.75g

Carbohydrate: 2g

Net Carbohydrates: 1.5g

Fiber: 0.5g

Protein: 11.5g

Keto Blueberry Chaffle

Preparation Time: 7 minutes

Cooking Time: 3 minutes

Servings: 2

Ingredients:

- 1 Egg (beaten)
- 1/2 cup of Mozzarella cheese (grated)
- 1 tsp. Erythritol
- 1/2 tsp. Baking powder
- 1 tsp. Blueberry extract
- 1/2 tsp. Cinnamon
- 12 Blueberries (fresh)

Directions:

1. Heat the mini-Chaffle maker with Cooking spray before ready to use.
2. Mix all of the ingredient*s in a bowl (except the blueberries). You should also use a mixer to mix the ingredients.
3. Pour ample batter into the Chaffle maker's middle and fan it out to the corners. If you overfill the first one, fill it up a little less every time to prevent spilling. 6 new blueberries on top
4. Allow 3 1/2 minutes to Cooking with the lid closed.

5. Remove the chaffle and set it aside to cool for 5 minutes on a cooling rack; repeat for the second chaffle. Add a dollop of whipped cream and a couple new blueberries on top.

Nutrition:

Calories: 121kcal

Carbohydrates: 3g

Protein: 9g

Fat: 8g

Cholesterol: 104mg

Sugar: 1g

The Best Ever Sweet Keto Chaffles

Preparation Time: 5 minutes

Cooking Time: 10-15 minutes

Servings: 3

Ingredients:

- 1 large egg
- 1/2 cup of shredded low moisture mozzarella
- 1/4 cup of almond flour
- 1/8 tsp. of gluten-free baking powder
- 3 tbsp. of granulated low-carb sweetener such as Erythritol or Swerve or brown sugar substitute
- Optional: pinch of cinnamon, vanilla / lemon zest

Directions:

1. To make the Chaffles, measure out all of the ingredients. Using a standard Chaffle maker to preheat a mini Chaffle maker.
2. You may either mix all of the ingredients together in a bowl or blend them together. In a mixer or food processor, mix the egg, mozzarella, almond flour, and baking powder.
3. After that, stir in the sweetener. The dough would be a bit runnier if the sweetener is added before mixing, so I like to add mine after.
4. Spoon one-third of the batter (3 to 4 tsp., around 55 g/1.9 oz.) into the hot Chaffle maker to produce three tiny Chaffles.

5. Cooking for 3 to 4 minutes with the Chaffle maker closed. In case the batter overflows, keep an eye on it (read our leak-proof tips above).

6. When you're done, remove the lid and set it aside to cool for a few moments. Transfer the chaffle to a cooling rack softly with a spatula. Continue for the remaining hitter.

7. Allow the chaffles to cool fully before serving. When they're hot, they'll be fluffy, but when they cool, they'll crisp up. Top with full-fat milk, coconut yogurt, whipped cream, bananas, and/or bacon syrup for a low-carb dessert. Serve with One-Minute Chocolate Milk, hot or cold!

8. Enjoy right away, or keep the chaffles in a sealed jar at room temperature for up to 3 days, or in the fridge for up to a week, without any toppings. The jar will hold them fluffy, but if you like them crispy, you can leave them out.

Nutrition

Calories 312

Fat 24

Carbohydrates 11.5

Sugar 0.8

Protein 11.6

Maple Pumpkin Keto Chaffle

Preparation Time5 minutes

Cooking Time16 minutes

Servings: 3

Ingredients:

- 2 eggs
- 3/4 tsp. baking powder
- 2 tsp. pumpkin puree
- 3/4 tsp. pumpkin pie spice
- 4 tsp. heavy whipping cream
- 2 tsp. Lakanto Sugar-Free Maple Syrup
- 1 tsp. coconut flour
- 1/2 cup of shredded mozzarella cheese
- 1/2 tsp. vanilla
- pinch of salt

Directions:

1. Chaffle or chaffle maker should be turned on. The Dash Mini Chaffle Maker is what I have.
2. Mix all ingredients in a small bowl.
3. 1/4 of the batter can be used to cover the dash mini Chaffle maker and Cook for 3-4 minutes.
4. Make 4 Maple Syrup Pumpkin Keto Chaffles by repeating the process three times more (Chaffles).
5. Serve with a dollop of sugar-free maple syrup or a scoop of keto ice cream.

Nutrition:

Calories: 201

Carbohydrates: 4g

Protein: 12g

Fat: 15g

Cholesterol: 200mg

Sodium: 249mg

Nut Butter Chaffle

Preparation Time5 minutes

Cooking 8 minutes

Servings: 2

Ingredients:

- 1 egg
- 1/2 cup mozzarella cheese, shredded
- 2 tablespoons almond flour
- 1/2 teaspoon baking powder
- 1 tablespoon sweetener
- 1 teaspoon vanilla
- 2 tablespoons nut butter

Directions:

1. Turn on the Chaffle maker.
2. Beat the egg in a bowl and combine with the cheese.
3. In another bowl, mix the almond flour, baking powder and sweetener.
4. In the third bowl, blend the vanilla extract and nut butter.
5. Gradually add the almond flour mixture into the egg mixture.
6. Then, stir in the vanilla extract.
7. Pour the batter into the Chaffle maker.
8. Cook for 4 minutes.
9. Set to a plate and let cool for 2 minutes.
10. Repeat the steps with the remaining batter.

Nutrition

Calories 168

Total Fat 15.5g

Saturated Fat 3.9g

Total Carbohydrate 1

Keto Coffee Chaffles

Preparation Time: 7 minutes

Cooking Time: 5 minutes

Servings: 2

Ingredients:

- 1 tbsp. almond flour
- 1 tbsp. instant coffee
- 1/2 cup cheddar cheese
- 1/2 tsp. baking powder
- 1 large egg

Directions:

1. Warmth Chaffle iron and grease with Cooking spray
2. Meanwhile, in a small mixing bowl, mix together all ingredients and 1/2 cup cheese.
3. Pour 1/8 cup cheese in a Chaffle maker and then pour the mixture in the center of greased Chaffle.
4. Again, sprinkle cheese on the batter.
5. Close the Chaffle maker.
6. Cooking chaffles for about 4-5 minutes until Cooked and crispy.
7. Once chaffles are cooked, remove and enjoy!

Nutrition

Protein: 26

Fat: 69

Chaffle Ice Cream Bowl

Preparation Time: 7 minutes

Cooking Time: 5 minutes

Servings: 2

Ingredients:

- 4 basic chaffles
- 2 scoops keto ice cream
- 2 teaspoons sugar-free chocolate syrup

Directions:

1. Arrange 2 basic chaffles in a bowl, following the contoured design of the bowl.
2. Top with the ice cream.
3. Drizzle with the syrup on top.
4. Serve.

Nutrition:

Calories 181

Total Fat 17.2g

Saturated Fat 4.2g

Cholesterol 26mg

Sodium 38mg

Total Carbohydrate 7g

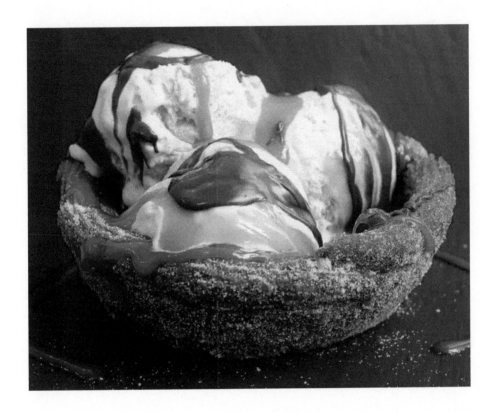

Scrambled Egg Stuffed Chaffles

Preparation Time: 7 minutes

Cooking Time: 28 minutes

Servings: 2

Ingredients:

For the chaffles:

- 1 cup finely grated cheddar cheese
- 2 eggs, beaten

For the egg stuffing:

- 1 tbsp. olive oil
- 1 small red bell pepper
- 4 large eggs
- 1 small green bell pepper
- Salt and ground black pepper
- 2 tbsp. grated Parmesan cheese

Directions:

For the chaffles:

1. Preheat the Chaffle iron.
2. In a medium bowl, mix the cheddar cheese and egg.
3. Open the iron; pour in a quarter of the mixture, close, and Cooking until crispy, 6 to 7 minutes.
4. Plate and make three more chaffles using the remaining mixture.

For the egg stuffing:

1. Meanwhile, warmth the olive oil in a medium skillet over medium heat on a stovetop.
2. In a medium bowl, beat the eggs with the bell peppers, salt, black pepper, and Parmesan cheese.
3. Pour the mixture into the skillet and scramble until set to your likeness, 2 minutes.
4. Between two chaffles, spoon half of the scrambled eggs and repeat with the second set of chaffles.
5. Serve afterward.

Nutrition

Calories 387

Fats 22.52g

Carbs 18

Net Carbs 17.52g

Protein 27.76g

Peanut Butter Sandwich Chaffle

Preparation Time: 7 minutes

Cooking Time: 5 minutes

Servings: 2

Ingredients:

For chaffle:

- 1 egg, lightly beaten
- 1/2 cup mozzarella cheese, shredded
- 1/4 tsp. espresso powder
- 1 tbsp. unsweetened chocolate chips
- 1 tbsp. Swerve
- 2 tbsp. unsweetened cocoa powder

For filling:

- 1 tbsp. butter, softened
- 2 tbsp. Swerve
- 3 tbsp. creamy peanut butter

Directions:

1. Preheat your Chaffle maker.
2. In a bowl, whisk together egg, espresso powder, chocolate chips, Swerve, and cocoa powder.
3. Add mozzarella cheese and stir well.
4. Spray Chaffle maker with Cooking spray.

5. Set 1/2 of the batter in the hot Chaffle maker and Cooking for 3-4 minutes or until golden brown. Repeat with the remaining batter.

6. For filling: In a small bowl, merge together butter, Swerve, and peanut butter until smooth.

7. Once chaffles is cool, then spread filling mixture between two chaffle and place in the fridge for 10 minutes.

8. Cut chaffle sandwich in half and serve.

Nutrition

Calories 1

Fat 16.1 g

Carbohydrates 9.6 g

Sugar 1.1 g

Protein 8.2 g

Cholesterol 101 mg

Chocolate Chaffle Rolls

Preparation Time: 7 minutes

Cooking Time: 10 minutes

Servings: 2

Ingredients:

- 1/2 cup mozzarella cheese
- 1 tbsp. almond flour
- 1 egg
- 1 tsp. cinnamon
- 1 tsp. stevia

Filling

- 1 tbsp. coconut cream
- 1 tbsp. coconut flour
- 1/4 cup keto chocolate chips

Directions:

1. Switch on a round Chaffle maker and let it heat up.
2. In a small bowl, merge together cheese, egg, flour, cinnamon powder, and stevia in a bowl.
3. Spray the round Chaffle maker with nonstick spray.
4. Pour the batter in a Chaffle maker and close the lid.
5. Close the Chaffle maker and Cooking for about 3-4 minutes.
6. Once chaffles are Cooked remove from Maker
7. Meanwhile, mix together cream flour and chocolate chips in bowl and microwave for 30 sec.
8. Spread this filling over chaffle and roll it.

9. Serve and enjoy!

Nutrition:

Protein: 32

Fat: 61

Carbohydrates: 7

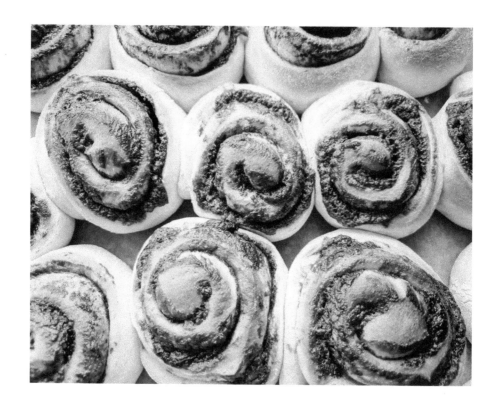

Lightning Source UK Ltd.
Milton Keynes UK
UKHW020647100621
385263UK00001B/107